The Blood Is!

Then There Are Bad Habits That Hinder Its Flow

Mable Nunley Dozier

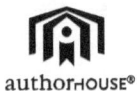

authorHOUSE®

AuthorHouse™
1663 Liberty Drive
Bloomington, IN 47403
www.authorhouse.com
Phone: 1-800-839-8640

First published by AuthorHouse 11/21/2011

ISBN: 978-1-4670-3967-3 (sc)
ISBN: 978-1-4670-3966-6(e)

Library of Congress Control Number: 2011917219

Printed in the United States of America

Any people depicted in stock imagery provided by Thinkstock are models, and such images are being used for illustrative purposes only.
Certain stock imagery © Thinkstock.

This book is printed on acid-free paper.

The Nunley Triplets

I dedicate this book to the triplets: R.C., A.V. and Mable Lee-they come in this order. We were known to be the first set of triplets born in West Tennessee. We were born in Martin, Tennessee on November 12, 1926. Now at the age of 85, we are thankful to God for many wonderful years of celebrating our birthdays together. We've celebrated every year together with the exception of my brother, who was in the Army for five years; so for 80 years we have had large family gatherings on our birthday. Thank God we are all still enjoying the time He has blessed us to have together!

And to the triplets born eighty three years later, cousins born in the same order boy, girl, boy. They are now two years old, living in Nashville IN.

BLOOD ABUSE

Blood abuse brings us to the awareness of bad habits that hinder the blood flow. Blood is our lifeline and the body becomes sick because of our bad habits. We should make the conscious decision to change all of our body's functions such as sleeping positions with our palms up and sitting upright. We should keep the body healing with good blood circulation. Practice, practice, practice!

Your Blood is Precious
Good habits can keep it flowing
Practice, practice, practice

Contents

Introduction   ix
Habits   1
Good Habits   2
Poor Circulation   6
Talk   11
As for Children   12
Telephone Survey   13
Questions   13
Food For Thought and the Body   14
Testimony   16
A Book of Poetry   17

Introduction

Man was created up right; to stand up right, to walk up right, to sit up right and to speak aright.

Aright is a word which means rightly, correctly. This is a word worth hearing but is not spoken often. Even in the dictionary there are only two words to define it: rightly and correctly.

The Biblical scriptures use the word aright only four times:
Psalm 50:23
"To him who orders his conduct aright, he will know
the salvation of God."
Psalm 78:8
"...a generation that did not set its heart aright."
Proverbs 15:2
"The tongue of the wise uses knowledge aright."
Jeremiah 8:6
"I listened and heard but they did not speak aright."

Written in a child like manner, this book will speak to the young and the adult alike. The goal is to show the natural powers of the human blood; if one would allow it to flow aright. The function of the human body has no respect of body. The blood must flow to be in good health. Each of us must listen and obey the laws of nature. We should learn to accept the need to change our life style habits. No one can change for you. We are all aware of how often words are repeated. We need to hear certain words over and over again in order to help us change our habits so our blood will flow properly and do its job of prevention and healing the body.

The key is to practice, practice, practice.

HABITS

Self control in your life and in your body is very important. The brain is the control center of the body. Every bodily function is operated by the brain but the blood is the power house of the body. The power of the blood provides wellness for the whole body. Man must have self control to have whole wellness. Life is habitual; there are good habits and bad habits. You will hear the word habit many times in this book to bring you in the awareness of your behavior. To change your bad habits into good habits start with focusing on one bad habit. Study the bad habit, listen to the body, what is it saying to you? Is your body comfortable, feeling a sense of joy, feeling good? Or, is your body in pain, some kind of discomfort? Be aware of your habits. Learn self control through practice, practice, practice.

Acceptance is the first step in changing your habits. Your habits are your own behavior; they are your own choices. Stop blaming others for the things you have decided to do to your own body! You have only one body so be good to yourself. Listen young people, middle-aged people and older people, it is never too late to accept change and to become healthy. Do it now!

Life is in the flow of the blood and without the blood there is no life. It flows from the waist up to the brain and from the waist down to the feet. Up or down habits cause so many health issues. All parts of the body suffer for the lack of circulation. The heart, Mr. Big, has become helpless because of bad habits

GOOD HABITS

In order to overcome your current bad habits, do not focus on the bad habits. You do need to be aware of those bad habits and call them out of your mind. Whatever is in the mind will be manifested and will take over your whole body. Once that happens bad habits turn into sickness. Stop now; become the master of your soul. Let the body be like an elephant. The elephant's master trains him to obey commands. The elephant obeys. As for you, obey the law of nature breaking the old bad habits. Remember, practice, practice, practice beginning with one bad habit and the others will follow! Yes, practice, practice, practice.

EATING

Do you sit up right as you eat? Probably not; this bad habit is so wide spread it seems enjoyable, even to die for. How much do you talk about eating? There is so much talk about eating. There are competitions about who can eat the most food. What good is this? We know the harm that can be done to the whole body from overeating and unhealthy eating, yet we continue in that bad habit. How do we eat? We eat very fast, filling our mouths with food, not chewing completely and it goes down causing stomach problems. As the food comes down it hinders the blood, poor circulation and then we just lay there wallowing in the food. We eventually come to a point where we then have to run to the doctor for all to be healed. With all of the attention in the media about healthy eating; no junk food, no sodas, drink more water - one would think that we would understand by now and make that change.

SITTING

This is another way we abuse our bodies. Listen with the mind to change the way these functions abuse the blood flow. Sitting can be so uncomfortable, but we have accepted the discomfort and continue sitting the same way complaining of the aches and pains from it. Don't slouch your shoulders or keep them unaligned with your ears. Don't lean forward. Try sitting upright with your back to the seat; almost immediately you will feel better. Now put your feet together and in line with your knees; not stretched out front or tucked in. Even in the bathroom you should sit upright (and everything will come out alright!). Practice, practice, practice; this will help you with self control – helping you to think of how you are sitting. Keep up the change and your blood will flow!

Sitting Exercise

Don't just flop down when you sit. Sit down with the thought of how to properly sit. Let the chair be upright as you relax. Place your feet flat on the floor with your legs straight. Avoid crossing your legs or ankles and no knee crossing. This will block the blood flow. Sit with your back to your seat. You will in time be in some discomfort or pain. Keep a relaxed mind and just practice, practice, practice. This is a good habit.

A Game

In a group, dinner party or church gathering give everyone ten toothpicks. Each time you see someone with their legs or arms crossed or not sitting upright, take one of their toothpicks. The one that collects the most toothpicks wins a prize. Practice, practice, practice.

STANDING

Some people just do not like to stand. It too can cause a lot of discomfort because of habit. There is no balance when you stand in certain ways. You see, balance is the key. There is such an unbalance with the whole body, so naturally standing improperly seems to be no big problem. It then becomes habit to stand that way and one does not even notice what is happening with the body. Once the pain comes – then off to the doctor for a quick fix!

Standing, walking or doing exercise without changing your behavior will not help. It only confirms that bad habits do affect blood flow which causes harm (pain) to the body. You think that by exercising you are helping but your shoulders are out of line with your head. Your knees are loose; have you ever thought about how your knees hold you up? When standing, lock your knees and they will bring you up right which will make you feel taller and your legs will support you with a new strength. That is standing upright. What is standing without the knees? In the bathroom, while brushing your teeth, do you stand with your legs apart with one turned one way or the other? When in the kitchen at the sink doing dishes how do you stand? The knees can not hold up under the pressure of the upper body without the mind of self control-putting the bad habits out of your mind.

Practice, practice, practice and you will become upright. Make a change and stand with your legs or your feet together. Stand properly and the knees will support, the upper body will be balanced and everything will work together. Try it, you might like it! Over time you will become aware of the good habit. Your mind and body will be working together; you will know the difference, you will feel the difference with practice, practice, practice. It may be uncomfortable at first, like beginning to exercise for the first time in a while. But you must be consistent and know you may prevent knee surgery. Sit upright with your feet together and knees in line with your legs. Your body and knees will work together. Practice, practice, practice.

Standing Exercise

Your total body will stand up with you by the law of nature. However, bad habits have taught the body to stand incorrectly. Stand up against a wall with your feet together. Your heels, your bottom, your shoulder blades and the back of your head should touch the wall. Do you feel that? That's what standing properly feels like. Practice, practice, practice.

What's Balance got to do With It?

Whole Wellness

Without balance one can not be upright. If one thing is off, it is like a boomerang. It throws the whole body off balance and it comes back to harm you.

Life Style of the Unbalanced

- Eating
- Water in take
- Finance
- Work
- Home
- Relationships
- Sexes
- God
- Love
- Standing
- Sitting
- Walking
- Sleeping
- Playing

One exhibits all of these bad habits in a day and this prevents the blood flow. Choose good habits or bad; which will it be?

Poor Circulation

Poor circulation is what happens when you abuse the blood flow. Walking will help with this problem. You are the only one who can walk for yourself!

1. Stop dragging yourself around.
2. Pick up your feet putting one down in front of the other.
3. Hold your head up and take deep breathes for proper oxygen in take.
4. Do not lean over while walking.
5. Trust yourself – you can walk upright.

Hands, legs, feet, knees and elbows are the trouble areas of the body because of their bending. It is happening all of the time; day and night. The joints are infection traps so be watchful of the bad habits and let the blood flow.

First let's deal with the legs. When you sit or lay it is highly likely that you have your legs crossed at some point during the day or night. The blood is truly trying to flow correctly and when it doesn't this causes cramps or pain. When this pain sets in and stays for periods of time, infection occurs and trouble starts. It's like the boomerang – you throw the bad habit out into your daily routine (crossing the legs) and now it's come back to harm you (pain and/or infection). This happens on all of the body's bending areas. However, bad habits can become good habits with practice, practice, practice.

WALKING

There are two kinds of walking: regular or normal paced walking and exercise or fast paced walking. To walk normally seems to be a struggle for some people as if they are "trying" to walk. Hold your head up and walk! Maybe to understand the struggle of some we should ask questions:

1. Does it hurt to walk?
2. How far can you walk?
3. Do you like to walk?
4. Does it hurt all over or just your feet?
5. What about your back or hips, are they in pain?

Think about how you should walk – the proper way to walk. Now, just walk with your head held up, shoulders back in line with the head and walk upright! Stay the course and walk wherever you are!

Exercise walking is structured walking. You have to do it properly for the exercise to benefit the body. When exercise walking, the body parts are all in proper line with the core and you walk at a fast pace causing the blood to pump by the movement of the arms and breathing in with the nostrils and out through the mouth. The head is up and the knees are bending. But when exercise is over…its right back to those bad habits, what happened?

Walking Exercise

When you need to move your body from one place to another, do so gracefully and with power. After you have mastered the sitting and standing exercises, proper walking will come naturally. Remember you are going somewhere and walking will get you there. You are in control by obeying the law of nature. Keep your head up and the other parts of your body will obey.

SLEEPING

Our bodies are wonderfully made. Why all of the health issues then? Habits, habits, habits – bad ones. It is never too late to go from bad to good. Remember, you are never too old to be in good health. Sleeping is to be in the unknown – unconscious; which is good because when the body is at rest the healing that is needed begins to take place from within as we are created to do. Because of the bad habits the healing that should be happening is being hindered. The body is all closed up. Your hand may be under your head which is stopping circulation. Your legs are crossed which is stopping circulation. Here are other examples of sleeping positions that hinder blood flow:

1. Laying your head on your hands
2. Knees are bent
3. Legs are crossed
4. Ankles are crossed
5. In the fetal position
6. Poor breathing habits
7. Lack of water
8. Eating late at night

These positions in which we sleep are slow killers. Because of bad habits people are dying in their sleep. Remember sleep is to be in the unknown – unconscious. Subconsciously your body moves into comfortable positions which are usually bad sleeping positions. Studies show that the best way to sleep is on your back. This takes total change to overcome the bad habits in your sleep pattern. It will take practice to change to this good habit, but to do so is quite wonderful for the circulation of your blood. Lay on your back with your legs straight, hands down by your side, no pillow. Pay attention, do you feel the blood flowing as it should? As soon as you feel yourself crossing, bending or tucking a body part move back to the proper position. To help practice this good habit, start by setting a goal of laying properly for 20 minutes then challenge yourself to do it longer and longer until now you have broken the bad habit! Of the twenty-four hours of a day, sleeping is the one thing we do longer than any other function. Take the time to rest and sleep well to be naturally healed by your blood flow. The body will go through three levels of sleep. The third level is when the brain starts the process of healing the body parts in need of repair. Practice, practice, practice. Here are some good sleeping habits to help you:

1. Have a special time to get into bed.
2. Sleep in a dark room.
3. No pillow (or a small one if you must).
4. Lie on your back and be as still as possible (this will give you control of your hands, legs and feet).
5. Do not dwell on anything – clear your mind.
6. Lay with your hands down by your side.
7. Trust your stillness; it is a good habit and good for you.
8. Plan to be consistent; it will heal your whole body.

This is only about you, your body and self control. At the end of each day the function of sleep takes over the whole body. Then, the new day comes in the morning to accept the change. As you progress in changing this bad habit to a good habit, other body functions will follow because the body works together. Heal thyself! Practice, practice, practice.

Sleeping Exercise

Take time during the day to lie on your back with your hands to your side and your feet up. Now pretend that you're standing up. Keep your arms and legs straight. This forces the blood to flow in the power of healing. Soon your body will be obeying the law of nature. This will become a good habit and your sleep will take on the three levels.

Hand and Feet Exercise

Use both hands in doing normal things like brushing your teeth or hair and ironing...everyday chores. While sitting, make circles with your feet and point them upward and down. Think exercise and do it!

THE HEAD

The head is the power over the whole body or the message center which sends whatever is in the mind to the rest of the body. Keep all bad habits out of your head. The good habits will not work with the bad ones. Usually there is something wrong in some other area of the body that is warning you to take notice to your behavior. Does your neck crack when you change position? Maybe the neck is feeling the weight of the head and not knowing how to deal with the blood abuse. Position your head when you move from one point to another. While sitting, what position is your head? Upright looking up and forward or is it down in your hands? When you are walking, is your head moving or bouncing around? Does your head feel heavy; too heavy to hold up? Take control and hold your head upright. Your head wants you to be in control. Listen to the body and take control and obey the law of nature for your health sake. Remain focused and hold your head up. Practice, practice, practice.

THE NECK

The neck is the junction of the head and the body connection. Do not allow things to linger there because it needs to be open to be free to let whatever passes flow and give nutrients and for liquids to go to the proper place for good health. Of course the neck holds the head in proper position. Don't allow your stubborn bad habits hinder the flow. Relax, do some neck rolls and be in self control. Be open to accept change and your neck will aid the whole body. Again, don't be stubborn, relax. Practice, practice, practice the good habits.

THE FACE

What is the face? It is what you want others to see. We are known by what other people see in our faces. Our behavior tells what is inside by what is seen on our faces. Therefore, if the blood is abused it shows up in the skin problems on our faces. The eyes also need a free flow of blood. As the old saying goes: "The eyes are the window to the soul". Do you know your face? Look in the mirror. Take care of your body and enjoy the beauty of your face. It is a reflection of happiness, hurt and pain. If there are bad habits, it shows first in the face; another form of blood abuse.

Don't hinder the flow of blood from the brain; it is the power of the whole body. Let go of the bad habits and practice, practice practice!

Talk

Be slow to speak about anything. This will give you time to think. That is to have self control rather than habitual speaking instead of sounding like it does not connect to you and your body. No one can talk for you. No one can use your mouth. Others can be supportive and with that support we will become confident in ourselves. We must encourage ourselves so that we will be able to be an example to others. That's a good habit.

Negative Expression Has Its Own Working Power
I can't
I'm trying
It's too hard
My nerves are bad
I hate this...I hate that
That is how I am
I am worried to death

Take control, and remember...As a man thinketh in his heart...so is he...

What does it all profit?

This is where the word aright is most important in our relationships. No man lives alone even if he wants to. Even if you have all the blood flowing and the body working together; what does it profit without conversation; aright conversation. This is right to know how to answer every man. Remember aright is without wrong. Practice using the word aright and it will become power within you. Practice, practice, practice.

*A Suggestion:
A Little Book Club*

1. Create a little book to track your changing behavior.
2. Make a new friend. Call two friends or a group of people and encourage each other.
3. Do a conference call for 20 or 30 minutes or text about your bad habits changing into good habits.
4. Use the little book to motivate your changing behavior and share with your group.
5. Be open-minded and honest with the group and with yourself.
6. Be consistent, have a set time that you call each other. For example every Tuesday at 8:30pm. Let it be important enough!!

As for Children

Children love story time. One way you can incorporate a healthier lifestyle, simplify a child's story time and make it fun is by reading the story and then ask questions. For example:

1. How long can you sit with your back to your seat?
2. How long can you hold your head up as you walk?
3. How long can you look into someone's eyes when you talk to them?

Make things even more fun by rewarding the child when they actually achieve those goals. Their young minds will receive and obey the law of nature. Practice, practice practice!

Telephone Survey

(The life style of the habits in three large cities)

- 80% from city to city has the same bad habits
- 90% in eating habits
- 70% in walking habits
- 80% in sleeping habits
- And on the average in all other body functions
- Just habit living!

Questions

1. What am I worried about?
2. What am I afraid of?
3. Why am I so stressful?
4. What about my relationships?
5. Do I really have faith?
6. Do I perform at my best on the job?
7. What is weighing me down?
8. What is it that is causing abuse to my body and blood?
9. Do I like myself?
10. Am I consumed by laziness?

Be honest, it hinders the blood flow when you're not.

Food For Thought and the Body

1. Good habits.
2. Sex! – Well…marriage is honorable.
3. Let nothing come between you and your blood.
4. Why not start now; love thy self.
5. Remember God is the greatest Love!!
6. Do you really want someone to take care of you? Would you really trust them?
7. Be free from the bondage of bad habits in all your ways.
8. Did someone make you angry or do you choose to be angry?
9. The condition of your body is because of what you've allowed.
10. The body is like a dead fish, with the blood flowing. Don't hinder its flow.
11. This awareness is a teacher. It's time to listen!
12. Marriage is honorable and the bed is not defiled, not a habit but a choice.
13. Lust is a **BIG** bad habit.
14. Habit is human behavior, good or bad.
15. What do you believe in?
16. If you could, would you change to do good all of the time?
17. What about lying; a real bad habit.
18. Reach out to someone and confess your bad habits to a brother or sister.
19. When you say, "I'll call you right back" and don't, that's lying; it's a bad habit.
20. Over eating and you're not hungry. That's a bad habit.

21. Just practice changing your bad habits to good habits.
22. Make new friends; sometimes it's easier to be open with people you don't know. Let yourself be free to newness and trust.
23. When you say you will do this or that, why not just do it?
24. If you lack knowledge you have no vision.
25. Blood abuse! Bad habit is an act of blood abuse.
26. Be honest with yourself; stop it now!!
27. Remember when you are sleeping lay on your back with arms and legs straight and loose. Lying on your side all curled up is shutting off the blood flow.
28. Why do you call people to talk about nothing?
29. Look now! Are your legs tucked back with your knees bent against your seat? Not good! That's a bad habit.

In conclusion, your blood is your life line. Make a good habit of whole wellness. Let it flow. Then there is the law of God. Make a good habit to let it flow; the blood of Jesus Christ. Seek and you shall find. No one can keep any law for you!!

For questions, for connecting with a believer, for support and to be supported call 904-768-9360 after 8:00pm.

Testimony

In 1984 or '85 I started having pains in my right leg. This continued for a week and a half. The pain was so severe, I could barely walk. I went to the doctor and discovered that I had a blood clot. I was immediately hospitalized for two weeks. During the course of my stay, I was constantly on my back with my leg propped up on a pillow. Since that time, I have slept on my back with arms at my side and my feet pointed upward, not knowing the benefits of this until I heard of this book. I have not had any problems with my legs in over 25 years and am so thankful to God for erasing my pain!

Brenda Dick
Atlanta, GA.

A Book of Poetry

MOVING FROM EYE TO EYE

From the natural to the all Seeing Eye! Here is a bit of poetry about the inner eye.

*"THE PLANK IN YOUR OWN EYE"

Take a look, my brother, within instead of looking out at others. For the plank in your eye is much bigger than the speck in your brother eye. Be filled with light for your brother to see, and your eye will see the light.

Let not the eye be evil. That means the eye is full of darkness and needs to see the light. The whole body is full of light, so set it on a stand for all to see.

*"IF THE EYE IS BAD"

What will you choose? Because of what you see, will the eye lead you astray because it's bad?

Now is the time to pluck it out and not be lost with two eyes, but saved with one.

* "THE ALL SEEING EYE"

I will guide you with my eye. You are the apple of my eye. I can change the darkness with the twinkling of my eye and then you will see me and be the light as I am the light.

* "EYE OF DARKNESS"

Can the eye of darkness see nothing but darkness and hope is no more? For there is no open door. How sad when no one in darkness can help because they too cannot see the open door. The door is not open because of the eye of darkness. Oh yes my brother! There is hope. Just turn around, for there is an open door and the all Seeing Eye is guiding you.

* "THE LAMP UNDER THE BASKET"

What a shame no one can see it. God said 'Let there be light'. The lamp is the eye watching you; not judging you, but guiding you with the light for you to see. It is not under the basket causing you to stumble in the darkness. Take heed. The all Seeing Eye is not under a basket, but is shining within you.

* "A SECRET PLACE"

Where is your lamp? Don't be deceived by your secret place. If your lamp is all about you, then it is under a basket. Put it on the lamp stand for others to see. The light that shines is from God above for you and I to see!

* "WHO IS THE ENEMY?"

Who or what is the enemy? The bad eye! Because of the bad eye there is no lamp. To be full of darkness is bad… bad! Turn around and seek the light The eye is there within. Just a little glimmer of light is power of the good eye; it is within you all the time. The body being full of light has no part with darkness.

* "HE HAS BLINDED THEIR EYES"

When your eye is good, the light can shine; but when your eye is bad, the heart is hardened. Open your eyes lest one should wait too late. So turn and see that the Lord can heal and set you free.

* "EYE FOR AN EYE, TOOTH FOR A TOOTH"

What profit is it to have your way? Remember, the all Seeing Eye is watching you. It sees you wherever you are. Your good eye is full of light. Let the light in to always shine for others to see Christ.

* "FACE TWO"

Take care of the whole body, but enjoy the beauty of the face! Let the blood flow and you will be healed.

*"IF THERE IS DARKNESS"

If you are in darkness, how great is the darkness? It is evil and very unhealthy and the whole body is sick. Christ is the Great Physician who heals and forgives. Now that you can see, stay in the light; the all Seeing Eye.

*"THE LAMP"

Take it everywhere you go. Let it shine, let it shine! Not only for you, but for all to see. Let it shine and keep it shining for the Kingdom's sake!

* "THE STRAIGHT WAY"

Let your eyes look straight ahead. Don't turn right or left. Remove your feet from evil. Pluck out your bad eye and stay in the narrow way. Let God wipe away all tears from your eyes, then the darkness will disappear forever. Stay in the light!

*"HOW FAR CAN YOU SEE?"

The eye goes deep and can see amazing things. Sometimes it is confused with what's not there. Now stop and look for the truth because the truth will not lie. The true light is the Lamb of God. Behold the Lamb!

Work Sheet Provided

Let Your Sleeping Position Be the First Focus
And the Other Habits Will Follow

A. List the changes you notice as you reveal them.

Take One Habit at a Time

A. Start with that one habit and work on it, to be healed

Healing Starts With a Changed Mind

A. List the desires you would like to change below

What Changes Have you Noticed?

A. List

Draw Some of Your Body Positions As They Are Now

Four (4) Weeks Later Draw Your Positions

What Are Your Positions

A. Name the positions as you become aware of them

Do You Sense Any Progress, Draw It Now

Keep a Record of the Beginning & End Results

A. List Below

Remember It All Starts in the Mind

A. List your thoughts

Are You Aware of Any Bad Habits

Such As:

A. Sleeping
B. Sitting
C .Walking
D. Standing
E. Eating

Keep The New Habit in Mind so you will continue to work on it

A. List

Now You Have Planted the Seed of Change

Make Notes When Necessary For Your Records

Make Notes When Necessary For Your Records

Make Notes When Necessary For Your Records